Put Your Weight loss in Overdrive

Put Your
Weight Loss in Overdrive

Benita and Jim Babeckis

Published for:
TRANZFORMATIONS
Oro Valley, Az. 85704

Email: Tranzform@Comcast.net
Website: http:// Tranzformations.net

Published for Tranzformations
8571 N. Calle Tioga
Oro Valley, Arizona 85704

ISBN No. 978-1440413322

Type composition and design by Full Moon Rising.
Cover illustration by Jim Babeckis - Graphic Design and Illustration.
Copyright © 2007. Cover design by Full Moon Rising

First Published October, 2008

Manufactured in the United States of America

Contents

Introduction

Evidence is mounting that a healthy diet can help protect you from some diseases. What you eat -- or don't eat -- may help prevent heart disease, cancer, osteoporosis and Type 2 diabetes.

With this in mind, here's how to use your diet to help reduce your risk of disease.

To help prevent heart disease, you need to keep your blood cholesterol, blood pressure and weight under control. Healthy eating habits can help you accomplish this, as well as reduce your risk for stroke.

Experts recommend these general nutrition goals for healthy adults:

* Your diet should include foods from all major foods groups, with special emphasis on fruits, vegetables and grains.

* Your diet should provide about 29 percent of daily calories from fat; only 10 percent of these fat calories should come from saturated fat. Trans fat should be 1 percent of daily calories or lower (trans fats are found in hydrogenated / partially hydrogenated vegetable oils).

* You should aim for at least five to thirteen servings (or 2-1/2 to 6-1/2 cups) of fruits andvegetables, depending on how many calories you need each day.

* You should aim for at least three servings equal to three ounces) a day of whole-grain foods.

* Choose fat-free and low-fat dairy products that are fortified with vitamin D over regular products.You should have three servings of these a day.

* Your protein should come from lean meats, poultry, fish and legumes with at least two servings of fish each week. Ten to thirty-five

*   percent of your daily calories should come
     from protein.

Other nutrition suggestions:

*   Choose fats and oils with two grams or less
     of saturated fat per tablespoon. These
     include liquid and tub margarines, canola oil
     and olive oil.

*   Limit the foods you eat that are high in
     calories or low in nutrition, such as soft
     drinks and candy.

*   Limit the amount of salt you eat each day to
     2,300 mg or less of sodium (equivalent to 5.8
     grams of salt).

*   Maintain your weight by balancing the
     number of calories you eat with the number
     that you use. Multiply the number of pounds
     you weigh by 15 calories. This represents the
     number of calories that you use in one day if
     you are moderately active. If you are mostly
     Sedentary, multiply your weight by 13
     instead of 15.

* Also maintain your weight by getting regular exercise for at least 30 to 60 minutes most days of the week.

* Limit your alcohol consumption to no more than two drinks a day if you are a man, or one a day if you are a woman or a man over the age of 65. One drink is equal to 12 ounces of beer, 4 ounces of wine and 1-1/2 ounces of 80-proof spirits.

Your diet should be low in sodium, saturated fat, cholesterol and total fat, as well as red meat, desserts and sugary beverages. Consume plenty of fruits, vegetables and low-fat dairy foods. Also include whole grains, poultry, fish and nuts. The typical American diet contains about 3,300 mg of sodium; the 2005 Dietary Guidelines Advisory Committee recommends that you eat no more than 2,300 mg a day.

To Combat Cancer

The best diet to help protect you against cancer helps you maintain a healthy weight and includes a variety of foods.

Obesity increases the risk for cancers of the endometrium (the lining of the uterus), colon, kidney, esophagus and breast (after menopause).

No single food is the perfect one for cancer prevention, but a combination of vitamins, minerals and phytochemicals (which come from plants) can offer good protection, according to the American Institute for Cancer Research (AICR).

Here are some examples of foods that researchers have identified as being particularly helpful in protecting against cancer:

* Green leafy vegetables such as spinach, kale, romaine lettuce and leaf lettuce contain fiber, folate and a variety of carotenoids, the AICR says. Carotenoids help prevent cancer by acting as antioxidants. The carotenoids in green leafy vegetables can help stop cell growth in cancers of the breast, skin, lung and stomach. Folate, too, may offer protection against Colorectal cancer, breast cancer and lung cancer.

* Cruciferous vegetables such as broccoli, cauliflower, cabbage and Brussels Sprouts contain substances that have been

associated with a lower risk for cancer, according to the AICR. They may help protect against cancers of the breast, endometrium, lung, colon, liver and cervix.

* Berries are good sources of vitamin C and fiber, but they also contain ellagic acid, which may help prevent cancers of the skin, bladder, lung, esophagus and breast, according to the AICR.

To help protect against cancer, your diet should include five to 13 servings of vegetables and fruits each day, according to the American Cancer Society (ACS) and the U.S. Department of Agriculture.

Here are some ways to add fruits and vegetables to your daily fare:

* Make sure vegetables and fruits are a part of every meal, and serve them as snacks.

* Limit the amount of fried vegetables you eat; prepare vegetables in healthier ways, such as by steaming or microwaving. Or eat them raw.
* If you want to drink fruit or vegetable juice, make sure it's 100 percent juice.

*   Other types of fruit beverages contain only small amounts of juice.

Besides fruits and vegetables, a healthy diet should include whole grains. Whole grains are rich in fiber, vitamins, minerals and a wide range of phytochemicals that may lower the risk for cancer, the AICR says.

You should choose whole grains over processed or refined grains and sugars. When buying rice, bread, pasta and cereal, look for varieties that are made from whole grains. The 2005 Dietary Guidelines Advisory Committee recommends that you eat at least 3 ounces of whole grains a day. Limit the amount of refined carbohydrates you eat. This includes pastries and desserts, sweetened cereals and soft drinks, according to the ACS.

When selecting sources of protein, choose fish, poultry or beans instead of beef, pork or lamb. When eating red meat, buy lean cuts and serve smaller portions. Bake, broil or poach meats instead of frying or grilling. This reduces the fat content.

Another food that may help protect against cancer is green tea. Both black tea and green tea contain polyphenols and flavonoids, which are antioxidants, according to the AICR. One type of flavonoid, catechins, seems particularly promising in its protective effect. Green tea contains about three times the amount of catechins that black tea has. Green tea may help protect against cancer of the colon, liver, breast and prostate.

To Fight Osteoporosis

The best step you can take against osteoporosis: Eat plenty of low-fat foods that are rich in calcium and fortified with vitamin D such as skim milk, low-fat yogurt and low-fat cheese, as well as broccoli.

Other steps you can take: Use calcium-fortified foods such as orange juice and breakfast cereals. Add soy foods, such as tofu and tempeh, to your diet. Besides being a good calcium source, soy foods have been shown to increase bone density. If you drink soy milk, buy brands that are calcium fortified.

Also, reduce your consumption of carbonated beverages. Studies show the phosphorus they contain may leech calcium from your bones. Not all carbonated beverages contain phosphorus, however. If "phosphoric acid" is not listed on the label, then the beverage will not affect your calcium levels.

Here are the recommended calcium intakes: Children ages 1 to 3 should get 500 mg of calcium each day; children ages 4 to 8 should get 800 mg; and children 9 to 12 should get 1,300 mg. Teens should consume 1,300 mg each day. Adults ages 19 to 50 should consume 1,000 mg each day; adults 50 and older should get 1,200 mg.

You should also make sure you get enough vitamin D in your diet and through exposure to sunlight, according to the National Osteoporosis Foundation (NOF). As we age, we are less able to make vitamin D through our skin.

That's why food sources of vitamin D become even more important in older adults. Good sources of vitamin D include fortified dairy products, egg yolks, ocean fish and liver. Most multivitamins and calcium supplements contain vitamin D.

You should get between 400 and 800 international units each day.

Do not take more than 800 IU a day unless your doctor prescribes it, because too much vitamin D may be harmful, the NOF says.

To Decrease Your Risk of Type 2 Diabetes

The best way to help prevent type 2 diabetes: Maintain a healthy weight by eating a balanced, low-fat diet. Obesity is a strong risk factor for developing type 2 diabetes.

Another strong risk factor for developing type 2 diabetes is having pre-diabetes, a condition in which your blood sugar is above normal, but not high enough to be diagnosed as diabetes. A person with pre-diabetes is at risk for developing type 2 diabetes within 10 years, and also is at higher risk for heart attack or stroke, according to the National Diabetes Education Program (NDEP), part of the National Institutes of Health.

Losing 5 to 7 percent of your weight if you are overweight can reduce your risk, according to the NDEP.

Other steps you can take to reduce your risk, according to the American Diabetes Association (ADA): Reduce your fat intake to less than 30 percent of your calories and your intake of saturated fat to less than 10 percent of your calories. Eat more high-fiber foods, such as oatmeal, beans, legumes, fresh fruits and fresh vegetables.

Get regular exercise, which help you with weight management, as well as reduce your risk. The USDA recommends 30 to 60 minutes of brisk walking or some other moderate exercise most days of the week to maintain your weight. To lose weight, 60 to 90 minutes a day may be needed.

Chapter 1:

Fat Burning Basics

If you're overweight, you are not a bad person. You're simply overweight. But it's important to lose the extra pounds so you'll look good, feel healthier and develop a sense of pride and self-esteem. Once you've lost the fat, you'll need to maintain your weight.

In this book you'll discover how to lose 10 pounds a month – a nice, safe loss of about two or two-and-a-half pounds a week – painlessly. You'll feel satisfied and more energetic than in the past without feeling deprived.

Most Americans pack on those extra pounds by eating the wrong things. Changing these poor eating habits is the key to long-term success. Knowledge – along with the right foods – is the key.

When humans lived in caves, they didn't know anything about preserving and storing food. They spent all their waking time and energy hunting and gathering food. When they had it, they ate it. Instead of storing food in pantries or cupboards, they stored energy in their bodies in the form of fat to burn during periods when there was little or nothing to eat.

Each year, it was absolutely vital for them to put on a good layer of fat during the warm spring and summer months. That was the only way they could guarantee their survival during the long and lean winter months. And since women bore the young, they needed more energy to sustain themselves and their babies, and that meant they were usually heavier.

Even though we no longer live in caves, we have inherited and maintained this basic mechanism for fat storage from our hunting and gathering ancestors. Each one of us is born with a certain number of fat cells. How many of these fat cells you possess depends on genetics. If you have a lot of fat cells, maybe your ancestors were the biggest people in the tribe, which was a good thing because they had the best chances of survival.

You can never get rid of fat cells, but – unfortunately – you can add to them. Depending upon what you eat, your body will manufacture new fat cells. And like those you were born with, they never go away. That doesn't mean you're doomed to be fat once you put on extra pounds. It is possible to shrink fat cells. That's what happens when you lose weight. You burn up the fat stored in those big fat cells. Think of them as balloons.

Burning off the fat inside them has the same effect as letting the air out of a balloon.

A good weight loss program requires a certain amount of intake restriction – the consumption of fewer calories. You burn off the fat by eating less fat and becoming more active.

To guarantee a lifetime of weight-control success, you have to change the type of foods you eat, so that you ingest less fat and still get the vitamins, minerals, trace elements, protein, and carbohydrates your body needs to thrive.

Extremely low-calorie diets may help you shed pounds quickly, but they'll lead to failure in the long run, because humans are genetically protected against starvation. During food shortages, our bodies slow down our metabolism and burn less energy so we can stay alive.

A part of our brain called the hypothalamus keeps us on an even weight keep by creating a "set point." That's the weight where we feel comfortable. The hypothalamus determines this point based on the level of consumption it's used to. It seeks to keep our weight constant, even if that point is over what it should be.

When we drastically cut back our food intake, the brain thinks the body is starving, and in an effort to preserve life, it slows the metabolism. Soon the pounds stop coming off. Consequently, we grow hungry and uncomfortable and then eat more. And then the diet fails.

How can you compensate for this metabolic slow-down? The answer is that you have to change the nutritional composition of the foods you eat. You will have to cut down on total calories – that's absolutely basic to weight loss.

More important, however, is reducing the percentage of total calories you are getting from fat. That's how you'll avoid starvation panic in your system. At the same time, you reduce the amount of fat in your food, replacing it with safe, low calorie, nutrient-rich plant foods. This will convince your brain that your body is getting all the nutrition it needs.

In fact, you'll be able to eat more food and feel more satisfied while consuming fewer calories and fats.

Plant foods break down slowly in your stomach, making you feel full longer, and they are rich in vitamins, minerals, trace elements, carbohydrates and protein for energy and muscle-building. This allows your body to burn off its excess stored fat.

Chapter 2:

Fat Burning Foods

Each one of the following foods is clinically proven to promote weight loss. These foods go a step beyond simply adding no fat to your system – they possess special properties that add zip to your system and help your body melt away unhealthy pounds. These incredible foods can suppress your appetite for junk food and keep your body running smoothly with clean fuel and efficient energy.

You can include these foods in any sensible weight-loss plan. They give your body the extra metabolic kick that it needs to shave off weight quickly.

A sensible weight loss plan calls for no fewer that 1,200 calories per day. However, Dr. Charles Klein recommends consuming more that that, if you can believe it – 1,500 to 1,800 calories per day. He says you will still lose weight quite effectively at that intake level without endangering your health.

Hunger is satisfied more completely by filling the stomach. Ounce for ounce, the foods listed below accomplish that better than any others. At the same time, they're rich in nutrients and possess special fat-melting talents.

Apples

These marvels of nature deserve their reputation for keeping the doctor away when you eat one a day. And now, it seems, they can help you melt the fat away, too.

First of all, they elevate your blood glucose (sugar) levels in a safe, gentle manner and keep them up longer than most foods. The practical effect of this is to leave you feeling satisfied longer, say researchers.

Secondly, they're one of the richest sources of soluble fiber in the supermarket. This type of fiber prevents hunger pangs by guarding against dangerous swings or drops in your blood sugar level, says Dr. James Anderson of the University of Kentucky's School of Medicine.

An average size apple provides only 81 calories and has no sodium, saturated fat or cholesterol. You'll also get the added health benefits of lowering the level of cholesterol already in your blood as well as lowering your blood pressure.

Eggs

Eggs are high in protein and essential to helping you burn fat. You may have heard all the warnings about eggs and health.That's because two eggs contain enough cholesterol to put you over the recommended amount of daily cholesterol intake. However, more recent studies have shown that dietary cholesterol has little effect on blood cholesterol. Dietary fat is the real culprit. That's the enemy that raises your bad cholesterol levels. If you're still concerned about your overall cholesterol intake, you can remove the yolk and still benefit from the high protein contained in eggs. Eggs contain the vitamin B-12 which is a key component in helping your body break down and burn fat.

Grapefruit

There's good reason for this traditional diet food to be a regular part of your diet. It helps dissolve fat and cholesterol, according to Dr. James Cerd of the University of Florida.

An average sized grapefruit has 74 calories, delivers a whopping 15 grams of pectin (the special fiber linked to lowering cholesterol and fat), is high in vitamin C and potassium and is free of fat and sodium. It's rich in natural galacturonic acid, which adds to its potency as a fat and cholesterol fighter. The additional benefit here is assistance in the battle against atherosclerosis (hardening of the arteries) and the development of heart disease.

Try sprinkling it with cinnamon rather than sugar to take away some of the tart taste.

All Citrus fruits like oranges, grapefruit, tangerines, lemons and limes contain high concentrations of Vitamin C (this is also called ascorbic acid). Vitamin C has a fat burning quality that reduces the effectiveness of fat. It reduces its content and can liquefy or dilute fat.

By diluting the fat, it makes it less effective and easier to flush out of your system. Vitamin C also works on cholesterol deposits. Vitamin C can help burn the cholesterol, hence making it difficult for cholesterol to form deposits in blood vessels.

Coffee

Easy does it is the password here. We've all heard about potential dangers of caffeine – including anxiety and insomnia – so moderation is the key. The caffeine in coffee can speed up the metabolism. In nutritional circles, it's known as a metabolic enhancer, according to Dr. Judith Stern of the University of California at Davis.

This makes sense, since caffeine is a stimulant. Studies show it can help you burn more calories than normal, perhaps up to 10 percent more. For safety's sake, it's best to limit your intake to a single cup in the morning and one in the afternoon. Add only skim milk to it and try doing without sugar – many people learn to love it that way. If you need a sweetener, **try Stevia.**

Mustard

Try the hot, spicy kind you find in Asian import stores, specialty shops and exotic groceries. Dr. Jaya Henry of Oxford Polytechnic Institute in England, found that the amount of hot mustard normally called for in Mexican, Indian and Asian recipes, about one teaspoon, temporarily speeds up the metabolism, just as caffeine and the drug ephedrine do.

"But mustard is natural and totally safe," Henry says. "It can be used every day, and it really works. We were shocked to discover it can speed up the metabolism by as much as 20 to 25 percent for several hours." This can result in the body burning an extra 45 calories for every 700 consumed, Dr. Henry says.

Oatmeal

While it may not be the tastiest thing you can eat, oatmeal definitely has some great nutritional qualities. You may have noticed that many of the oatmeal brands are now boasting that eating more oatmeal will help lower your cholesterol level. That's because oatmeal is loaded with soluble fiber which helps reduce blood cholesterol by flushing those bad digestive acids out of your system.

The best kind of oatmeal to eat is unsweetened and unflavored. While I know it's tempting to select the apples and cinnamon flavor and load it with butter and sugar -- you really lose out on all the health benefits.

If you must sweeten your bowl of oatmeal, do so by adding fruit. We prepare ours with a handful of fruit (much better for you than sugar) Oatmeal is also beneficial in fighting colon cancer and heart disease.

Olive Oil

Certain fats are good for you and your body needs them. Olive oil is one of those "good fats". In fact, it's so good that it helps you burn fat and keeps your cholesterol down. Olive oil is rich in monounsaturated fat, a type of fat that researchers are finding provide outstanding health benefits. One ounce of extra virgin olive oil contains about 85% of the daily value for monounsaturated fat. So instead of taking a swig of orange juice in the morning, many dieters are picking up a bottle of extra virgin olive oil.

Peppers

Hot, spicy chili peppers fall into the same category as hot mustard, Henry says.

He studied them under the same circumstances as the mustard and they worked just as well. A mere three grams of chili peppers were added to a meal consisting of 766 total calories. The peppers' metabolism-raising properties worked like a charm, leading to what Henry calls a diet-induced thermic effect. It doesn't take much to create the effect. Most salsa recipes call for four to eight chilies – that's not a lot. Peppers are astonishingly rich in vitamins A and C, abundant in calcium, phosphorus, iron and magnesium, high in fiber, free of fat, low in sodium and have just 24 calories per cup.

Potatoes

We've got to be kidding, right? Wrong. Potatoes have developed the same "fattening" rap as bread, and it's unfair. Dr. John McDougal, director of the nutritional medicine clinic at St. Helena Hospital in Deer Park, California, says, "An excellent food with which to achieve rapid weight loss is the potato, at 0.6 calories per gram or about 85 calories per potato." A great source of fiber and potassium, they lower cholesterol and protect against strokes and heart disease.

Preparation and toppings are crucial. Steer clear of butter, milk and sour cream, or you'll blow it. Opt for yogurt instead.

Rice

An entire weight-loss plan, simple called the Rice Diet, was developed by Dr. William Kempner at Duke University in Durham, North Carolina. The diet, dating to the 1930's, makes rice the staple of your food intake. Later on, you gradually mix in various fruits and vegetables. It produces stunning weight loss and medical results. The diet has been shown to reverse and cure kidney ailments and high blood pressure.

A cup of cooked rice (150 grams) contains about 178 calories – approximately one-third the number of calories found in an equivalent amount of beef or cheese. And remember, whole grain rice is much better for you than white rice.

Soups

Soup is good for you! Maybe not the canned varieties from the store – but old-fashioned, homemade, soup promotes weight loss. A study by Dr. John Foreyt of Baylor College of Medicine in Houston, Texas, found that dieters who ate a bowl of soup before lunch and dinner lost more weight than dieters who didn't. In fact, the more soup they ate, the more weight they lost. And soup eaters tend to keep the weight off longer. Naturally, the type of soup you eat makes a difference. Cream soups or those made of beef or pork are not your best bets. But here's a great recipe:

Slice three large onions, three carrots, four stalks of celery, one zucchini and one yellow squash. Place in a kettle. Add three cans crushed tomatoes, two packets low-sodium chicken bouillon, three cans water and one cup white wine (optional). Add tarragon, basil, oregano, thyme and garlic powder. Boil, then simmer for an hour. Serves six.

Spinach

Popeye really knew what he was talking about, according to Dr. Richard Shekelle, an epidemiologist at the University of Texas. Spinach has the ability to lower cholesterol, rev up the metabolism and burn away fat. Rich in iron, beta carotene and vitamins C and E, it supplies most of the nutrients you need.

Tofu

You just can't say enough about this health food from Asia. Also called soybean curd, it's basically tasteless, so any spice or flavoring you add blends with it nicely. A 2½ " square has 86 calories and nine grams of protein. (Experts suggest an intake of about 40 grams per day.) Tofu contains calcium and iron, almost no sodium and not a bit of saturated fat. It makes your metabolism run on high and even lowers cholesterol. With different varieties available, the firmer tofu are good for stir-frying or adding to soups and sauces while the softer ones are good for mashing, chopping and adding to salads.

Whole Grains (and Bread)

These days everyone seems to be screaming "No carbs!" It's as if the world has gone no-carb crazy and everyone is running from sliced breads and pastas. Well the truth is, your body needs carbohydrates. If you go without them completely your body will start to crave them. So it's not a good idea to exclude all carbs because the right kinds are actually good for you.

It's the processed carbohydrates that are bad for you -- the white breads, bagels, pastas, and white rice to name a few.

None of the above foods come out of the ground the way you eat them, which is usually a bad sign. They've all been processed, thus stripping out all the nutrients leaving you with loads of starch. The key is to eat "whole grain" foods because they haven't been processed and contain the fiber and minerals your body needs. So don't be fooled by a loaf of bread labeled "wheat". Regular wheat bread is still lacking in vitamins and minerals. Manufacturers add molasses to it so it turns brown. Don't let them trick you. The only kind of bread that's good for you is the kind that's labeled "whole grain".

You needn't dread bread. It's the butter, margarine or cream cheese you put on it that's fattening, not the bread itself. We'll say this as often as needed — fat is fattening. If you don't believe that, ponder this — a gram of carbohydrate has four calories, a gram of protein four, and a gram of fat nine. So which of these is really fattening?

Bread, a natural source of fiber and complex carbohydrates, is okay for dieting. Norwegian scientist Dr. Bjarne Jacobsen found that people who eat less than two slices of bread daily weigh about 11 pounds more that those who eat a lot of bread.

Studies at Michigan State University show some breads actually reduce the appetite. Researchers compared white bread to dark, high-fiber bread and found that students who ate 12 slices a day of the dark, high-fiber bread felt less hungry on a daily basis and lost five pounds in two months.

Others who ate white bread stayed hungrier, ate more fattening foods and lost no weight during this time. So the key is eating dark, rich, high-fiber breads such as pumpernickel, whole wheat, mixed grain, oatmeal and others.

The average slice of whole grain bread contains only 60 to 70 calories, is rich in complex carbohydrates – the best, steadiest fuel you can give your body – and delivers surprising amount of protein.

Chapter 3:

Super Foods

It would be unrealistic to think you could successfully lose weight and enjoy what you're eating with a mere handful of foods, no matter how delicious, nutritious and satisfying they may be. So we're going to add an extra roster of fat-fighting foods you can eat along with the great foods mentioned in the last section.

They'll lend different tastes and textures to every meal and provide a wide range of vitamins, minerals, proteins and other vital nutrients. Naturally, each one is high in fiber, low in fat and safe when it comes to sodium content, too.

Many have crunchiness and flavor we've come to desire in snack and nibbling foods. If you're like most of us, you may have a real junk food snacking habit – a habit you're going to have to change in order to slim down. Many of the foods in this section may be worthy substitutes.

Asparagus

Asparagus contains the chemical asparagines. This is an alkaloid that stimulates the kidneys and improves the circulatory process. These alkaloids directly affect the cells and break down fat. They also contain a chemical that helps remove waste from the body by breaking up the oxalic acid (this acid tends to glue fat to cells so breaking the acid up helps to reduce fat levels).

Barley

This filling grain stacks up favorably to rice and potatoes. It has 170 calories per cooked cup, respectable levels of protein and fiber and relatively low fat. Roman gladiators ate this grain regularly for strength and actually complained when they had to eat meat.

Studies at the University of Wisconsin show that barley effectively lowers cholesterol by up to 15%. It also contains powerful anti-cancer agents. Israeli scientists say it cures constipation better than laxatives - and can promote weight loss, too. Use it as a substitute for rice in salads, pilaf or stuffing, or add to soups and stews. You can also mix it with rice for an interesting texture. Ground into flour, it makes excellent breads and muffins.

Beans

While beans are often associated with the gastrointestinal disturbances they may cause, they are also very good sources of protein, fiber and iron.

Some of the best kinds of beans to eat are:

* Navy beans
* White beans
* Kidney beans
* Lima beans

And as always, there are those beans that you should limit in your diet – We're talking about those that are baked and refried. Refried beans contain tons of saturated fat while baked beans are usually loaded in sugar. Sure, you'll be getting your protein but you'll also be consuming a lot of fat and sugar you don't need. Here's something else to remember.

Be sure to cook your beans thoroughly because our digestive tracks are not adapted to breaking down some proteins that are contained in certain beans. They are already good enough on their own at stimulating GI activity. You don't want to create any unnecessary turbulence in your tummy)

Tip: Edamame (pronounced ed-uh-ma-may) is an organic soybean in a pod often served at Japanese restaurants. All you do is boil them for three minutes, add a pinch of salt and eat the soybeans out of the pods. They are surprisingly tasty and very good for you. One serving contains 10 grams of soy protein. The best place to find them is at a store that sells organic foods. (Whole Foods, for example).

Beans are one of the best sources of plant protein. Peas, beans and chickpeas are collectively known as legumes. Most common beans have 215 calories per cooked cup (lima beans go up to 260). They have the most protein with the least fat of any food, and they're high in potassium but low in sodium. Plant protein is incomplete, which means that you need to add something to make it complete. Combine beans with a whole grain – rice, barley, wheat, corn – to provide the amino acids necessary to form a complete protein. Then you get the same top-quality protein as in meat with just a fraction of the fat. Studies at the University of Kentucky and in the Netherlands show that eating beans regularly can lower cholesterol levels.

The most common complaint about beans is that they cause gas.

Here's how to contain that problem, according to the U.S. Department of Agriculture (USDA): Before cooking, rinse the beans and remove foreign particles, put in a kettle and cover with boiling water, soak for four hours or longer, remove any beans that float to the top, then cook the beans in fresh water.

Beets

Beets are a strong diuretic that focuses on the liver and kidneys. Beets flush out floating body fats. They have a special iron that cleanses the corpuscles, corpuscles are blood cells that can contain fatty deposits. It also contains a chlorine that also helps to flush out fatty deposits. This chlorine stimulates the lymph which will clear out the fat deposits.

Beets are a strong diuretic that focuses on the liver and kidneys. Beets flush out floating body fats. They have a special iron that cleanses the corpuscles. Corpuscles are blood cells that can contain fat deposits.

Berries

These are the perfect weight-loss food. Berries have natural fructose sugar that satisfies your longing for sweets and enough fiber so you absorb fewer calories that you eat. British researchers found that the high content of insoluble fiber in fruits, vegetables and whole grains reduces the absorption of calories from foods enough to promote width loss without hampering nutrition.

Berries are a great source of potassium that can assist you in blood pressure control. Blackberries have 74 calories per cup, blueberries 81, raspberries 60 and strawberries 45. So use your imagination and enjoy the berry of your choice.

Broccoli

Broccoli is America's favorite vegetable, according to a recent poll. No wonder. A cup of cooked broccoli has a mere 44 calories.

It delivers a staggering nutritional payload and is considered the number one cancer-fighting vegetable. It has no fat, loads of fiber, cancer fighting chemicals called indoles, carotene, twenty-one times the RDA of vitamin C and calcium.

When buying broccoli, pay attention to the color. The tiny florets should be rich green and free of yellowing. Stems should be firm.

Brussels Sprouts

This vegetable stimulates the glands, especially the pancreas, which releases hormones that have a cleansing affect on cells. They also contain minerals that stimulate the kidneys. Waste is released quicker and that helps to clean out the cells.

Buckwheat

It's great for pancakes, breads, cereal, soups or alone as a grain dish commonly called kasha. It has 155 calories per cooked cup. Research at the All India Institute of Medical Sciences shows diets including buckwheat lead to excellent blood sugar regulation, resistance to diabetes and lowered cholesterol levels.

You cook buckwheat the same way you would rice or barley. Bring two to three cups of water to a boil, add the grain, cover the pan, turn down the heat and simmer for 20 minutes or until the water is absorbed.

Cabbage

This Eastern Europe staple is a true wonder food. There are only 33 calories in a cup of cooked shredded cabbage, and it retains all its nutritional goodness no matter how long you cook it. Eating cabbage raw (18 calories per shredded cup), cooked, as sauerkraut (27 calories per drained cup) or coleslaw (calories depend on dressing) only once a week is enough to protect against colon cancer.

Surveys in the United States, Greece and Japan show that people who eat a lot of it have the least colon cancer and the lowest death rates overall.

Carrots

What list of health-promoting, fat-fighting foods would be complete without Bugs Bunny's favorite? A medium-sized carrot carries about 55 calories and is a nutritional powerhouse. The orange color comes from beta carotene, a powerful cancer-preventing nutrient (provitamin A). Chop and toss them with pasta, grate them into rice or add them to a stir-fry. Combine them with parsnips, oranges, raisins, lemon juice, chicken, potatoes, broccoli or lamb to create flavorful dishes.

Spice them with tarragon, dill, cinnamon or nutmeg. Add finely chopped carrots to soups and spaghetti sauce – they impart a natural sweetness without adding sugar.

Celery

Raw celery has a high concentration of Calcium in a ready to use form so when you eat it, the calcium is sent directly to work. This pure form of calcium will ignite your endocrine system. The hormones in your body will break up the accumulated fat build ups. Celery also has a high level of magnesium and iron which will clean out your system.

Chicken

White meat contains 245 calories per four ounce serving and dark meat, 285. It's an excellent source of protein, iron, niacin and zinc. Skinned chicken is healthiest, but most experts recommend waiting until after cooking to remove it because the skin keeps the meat moist during cooking.

Corn

It's really a grain – not a vegetable – and is another food that's gotten a bum rap. People think it has little to offer nutritionally and that just isn't so. There are 178 calories in a cup of cooked kernels.

It contains good amounts of iron, zinc and potassium, and University of Nebraska researchers say it delivers a high-quality of protein, too.

The Tarahumara Indians of Mexico eat corn, beans and hardly anything else. Virgil Brown, M.D., of Mount Sinai School of Medicine in New York, points out that high blood cholesterol and cardiovascular heart disease are almost nonexistent among them.

Cucumber

Cucumbers have high sulphur and silicon content. These minerals work to stimulate the kidneys to wash out uric acid which is a waste product. With uric acid being washed out, the removal of fat is stimulated. Fat is also loosened from cells.

Cottage Cheese

As long as we're talking about losing weight and fat-fighting foods, we had to mention cottage cheese. Low-fat (2%) cottage cheese has 205 calories per cup and is admirably low in fat, while providing respectable amounts of calcium and the B vitamin riboflavin. Season with spices such a dill, or garden fresh vegetable such a scallions and chives for extra zip. To make it sweeter, add raisins or one of the fruit spreads with no sugar added.

You can also use cottage cheese in cooking, baking, fillings and dips where you would otherwise use sour cream or cream cheese.

Figs

Fiber-rich figs are low in calories at 37 per medium (2.25" diameter) raw fig and 48 per dried fig. A recent study by the USDA demonstrated that they contribute to a feeling of fullness and prevent overeating.

Subjects actually complained of being asked to eat too much food when fed a diet containing more figs than a similar diet with an identical number of calories. Serve them with other fruits and cheeses. Or poach them in fruit juice and serve them warm or cold. You can stuff them with mild white cheese or puree them to use as a filling for cookies and low-calorie pastries.

Fish and Seafood

The health benefits of fish are greater than experts imagined – and they've always considered it a health food. The calorie count in the average four-ounce serving of a deep-sea fish runs from a low of 90 calories in abalone to a high of 236 in herring. Water-packed tuna, for example, has 154 calories. It's hard to gain weight eating seafood.

As far back as 1985, articles in the New England Journal of Medicine showed a clear link between eating fish regularly and lower rates of heart disease. The reason is that oils in fish thin the blood, reduce blood pressure and lower cholesterol.

Dr. Joel Kremer, at Albany Medical College in New York, discovered that daily supplements of fish oil brought dramatic relief to the inflammation and stiff joints of rheumatoid arthritis.

Greens

We're talking collard, chicory, beet, kale, mustard, Swiss chard and turnip greens. They all belong to the same family as spinach, and that's one of the superstars. No matter how hard you try, you can't load a cup of plain cooked greens with any more than 50 calories. They're full of fiber, loaded with vitamins A and C, and free of fat. You can use them in salads, soups, casseroles or any dish where you would normally use spinach.

Horseradish

We've all seen horseradish but few venture to use it. Horseradish has the amazing effect of dissolving fat in cells (no side effects) and also has a cleansing effect on the body.

Kiwi

This New Zealand native is a sweet treat at only 46 calories per fruit. Chinese public health officials praise the tasty fruit for its high vitamin C content and potassium. It stores easily in the refrigerator for up to a month. Most people like it peeled, but the fuzzy skin is also edible.

Leeks

These members of the onion family look like giant scallions, and are every bit as healthful and flavorful as their better-known cousins. They come as close to calorie-free as it gets at a mere 32 calories per cooked cup. You can poach or broil halved leeks and then marinate them in vinaigrette or season with Romano cheese, fine mustard or herbs. They also make a good soup.

Lettuce

People think lettuce is nutritionally worthless, but nothing could be farther from the truth. You can't leave it out of your weight-loss plans, not at 10 calories per cup of raw romaine. It provides a lot of filling bulk for so few calories.

And it's full of vitamin C, too. Go beyond iceberg lettuce with Boston, Bib and Cos varieties or try watercress, arugula, radicchio, dandelion greens, purslane and even parsley to liven up your salads

Melons

Now, here's great taste and great nutrition in a low-calorie package! One cup of cantaloupe balls has 62 calories, on cup of casaba balls has 44 calories, one cup of honeydew balls has 62 calories and one cup of watermelon balls has 49 calories. They have some of the highest fiber content of any food and are delicious. Throw in handsome quantities of vitamins A and C plus a whopping 547 mgs of potassium in that cup of cantaloupe, and you have a fat-burning health food beyond compare.

Oats

A cup of oatmeal or oat bran has only 110 calories. And oats help you lose weight. Subjects in Dr. James Anderson's landmark 12-year study at the University of Kentucky lost three pounds in two months simply by adding 100 grams (3.5 ounces) of oat bran to their daily food intake and nothing else.

Onions

Flavorful, aromatic, inexpensive and low in calories, onions deserve a regular place in your diet. One cup of chopped raw onions has only 60 calories, and one raw medium onion (2.15" diameter) has just 42. They control cholesterol, thin the blood, and may have some value in counteracting allergic reactions. Most of all, onions taste good and they're good for you.

Partially boil, peel and bake, basting with olive oil and lemon juice. Or sauté them in white wine and basil, then spread over pizza. Or roast them in sherry and serve over paste.

Pasta

The Italians had it right all along. A cup of cooked paste (without a heavy sauce) has only 155 calories and fits the description of a perfect starch-centered staple. Analysis at the American Institute of Baking shows pasta is rich in six minerals, including manganese, iron, phosphorus, copper, magnesium and zinc. Also be sure to consider whole wheat pastas, which are even healthier.

Sweet Potatoes

You can make a meal out of them and not worry about gaining a pound – and you sure won't walk away from the table feeling hungry. Each sweet potato has about 103 calories. Their creamy orange flesh is one of the best sources of vitamin A you can consume.

You can bake, steam or microwave them. Or add them to casseroles, soups and many other dishes. Flavor with lemon juice or vegetable broth instead of butter.

Tomatoes

A medium tomato (2.5" diameter) has only about 25 calories. These garden delights are low in fat and sodium, high in potassium and rich in fiber. A survey at Harvard Medical School found that the chances of dying of cancer are lowest among people who eat tomatoes (or strawberries) every week. And don't overlook canned crushed, peeled, whole or stewed tomatoes. They make sauces, casseroles and soups taste great while retaining their nutritional goodness and low-calorie status. Even plain old spaghetti sauce is a fat-burning bargain when served over pasta, so think about introducing tomatoes into your diet

Turkey and Lean Meats

Turkey and beef are great for building muscle and boosting the immune system, but as always you have to be careful: Basted turkeys are usually injected with fatty substances while beef contains saturated fat. So while, you might give thanks to those pilgrims for starting the wonderful tradition of Thanksgiving turkey. It just so happens that this health food disguised as meat is good year-round for weight control.

A four-ounce serving of roasted white meat turkey has 177 calories and dark meat has 211. Sadly, many folks are still unaware of the versatility and flavor of ground turkey. Anything hamburger can do, ground turkey can do at least as well, from conventional burgers to spaghetti sauce to meat loaf. Some ground turkey contains skin which slightly increases the fat content. If you want to keep it really lean, opt for ground breast meat. But since this has no added fat, you'll need to add filler to make burgers or meat loaf hold together. Buying turkey has become easy. It's no longer necessary to buy a whole bird unless you want to.

Ground turkey is available fresh or frozen, as are individual parts of the bird, including drumsticks, thighs, breasts and cutlets. And if you are going to eat beef, be sure to consume the leanest cuts you can find by looking for "loin" or "round" on the labels.

Salmon and tuna are also good sources of protein. They both contain omega-3 fatty acids which may sound bad, but are actually healthy fats. These two foods are also good for giving your immune system a nice boost and should be consumed at least 3 times a week.

It's not only about what you eat, but how and when you eat. Your eating habits play a vital role in how your body burns fat.

It's not only about what you eat, but how and when you eat. Your eating habits play a vital role in how your body burns fat.

Yogurt

The non-fat variety of plain yogurt has 120 calories per cup and low-fat, 144. It delivers a lot of protein and, like any dairy food, is rich in calcium and contains zinc and riboflavin.

Yogurt is handy as a breakfast food – cut a banana into it and add the cereal of your choice. You can find ways to use it in other types of cooking, to – sauces, soups, dips, toppings, stuffing and spreads. Many kitchen gadget departments even sell a simple funnel for making yogurt cheese. Yogurt can replace heavy creams and whole milk in a wide range of dishes, saving scads of fat and calories.

You can substitute half or all of the higher fat ingredients. Be creative. For example, combine yogurt, garlic powder, lemon juice, a dash of pepper and Worcestershire sauce and use it to top a baked potato instead of piling on fat-laden sour cream. According to an article in Obesity Research, women who ate low-fat dairy products, such as nonfat yogurt and low-fat milk, three to four times a day lost 70 percent more fat than low-dairy dieters. In another study done at Purdue University those who consumed 3 cups of fat-free milk gained less weight over the course of 2 years than those on low calcium diets. So, not only do dairy products help you strengthen your bones, they can also play an essential role in burning that unwanted body fat. If you are a regular consumer of milk and other dairy products, that's great (as long as you don't overdo it). Just watch your proportions and perhaps switch over to the low or no fat varieties.

Supermarkets and health food stores sell a variety of yogurts, many with added fruit and sugar. To control calories and fat content, buy plain non-fat yogurt and add fruit yourself. Apple butter or fruit spreads with little or no added sugar are an excellent way to turn plain yogurt into a delectable sweet treat.

Chapter 4:

Some Things to Keep in Mind During Weight loss

Eat breakfast within an hour of rising.

During the night, your metabolism slows down. To get it going again, you need to eat something.

It's better to eat smaller meals more often than only three medium to large meals a day.

Eating more frequently will prevent you from feeling hungry, throughout the day. And if you're eating fiber and protein and drinking enough water, you will actually feel fuller for longer periods and not have the urge to snack as much.

The key to slimming down is not to eat less, just eat more sensibly.

We know it sounds funny but it's true. The actual process of digestion burns up calories. So if you eat several meals throughout the day, you'll burn up more calories.

Stop Eating 3 Hours Before Bedtime

You've probably seen the suggestion of not eating anything after 7 pm. Well this generally assumes you go to bed around 9 or 10 at night. If you are a night owl, you may retire a little later so it may seem unrealistic to not eat anything after 7 if you don't go to bed until 12 am Generally, the rule of the thumb is to not eat anything within 3 hours of your bedtime. So if you do usually go to sleep at 1 am. this would mean no food intake after 10 pm. The reason you don't want to eat late at night is because your food may not properly digest. This can cause morning gas and stomach cramps. Some people who complain about bloating never realize that it's from the gas and food particles left over from improper digestion. This can be avoided if you cut down the late night snacking.

Eating late at night also forces your body to use its energy on digestion. One of the primary functions of sleep is to help you recuperate from the day. You want your body to be as relaxed as possible so you can wake up energized.

Now we all know we have to cheat at some points. It's just not realistic to believe you can refrain from eating late at night every single night. So if you must cheat, then eat something healthy like a piece of fruit or a very small handful of nuts.

Stop Emotional Eating

This is probably easier said than done for most people. If you are stressed, depressed or lacking emotional support from friends, family or loved ones you may resort to emotional eating. This is a terrible eating habit because it causes you to eat between meals and when you're not hungry. Sometimes you may think you are a hungry but in reality you may just be lonely and are using food to comfort you and fill a void. Stress and depression also causes an increase production of the hormone cortisol and can also add more tummy fat.

If this is a problem for you, it's important to seek help from either a professional, church members, friends or family. One thing is for sure...stress and flat stomachs are like oil and water. They just don't mix.

Cut Down on Sodium (Salt)

Sodium can cause lots of bloating and make your tummy actually look flabbier than it really is. Be careful...a lot of people associate sodium with foods that taste salty. This can get tricky because sodium is in all kinds of foods. Manufacturers use tons of it for preservation. Almost all canned foods, TV dinners and those soup-to-go lunches are the worst! Have you ever read those labels? Some of them contain over half of your daily intake! We've found that the best TV dinners are the "Smart Ones" brand.

Smart Ones still contain 25% of your daily intake of salt. That's pretty high for one serving but it's much better than some of the other brands.

When trying to lose weight, a lot of people forget to watch what they drink or the kind of salad dressing they put on their salads - in other words, the little things. All these things add up and can hinder weight loss, so we wrote a book about it. This is it.

Analyze Your Habits

Now it's time to think about your own eating habits. Are you eating breakfast every morning within one hour of rising? Are you snacking between meals? And if so, what kinds of snacks are you eating? If you do get the urge to snack between your meals, make healthier choices like fruits and vegetables.

Remember, you can jazz up your snacks. Instead of eating a plain apple, try adding a teaspoon of peanut butter to enhance the taste. You'll be getting additional protein as well. Spice up your plain carrot sticks by adding a small amount of low-fat vegetable dip for more flavor.

Now it's time to for you to evaluate your own habits and decide where they need improvement.

Remember...eat healthy, eat often.

Chapter 5:

Healthy Snacks

Popcorn

As long as you don't saturate it in butter and/or salt (a.k.a. movie theatre popcorn) this is a very healthy snack. It's very high in fiber and low in calories. The best kind to eat is the air popped but if you're going to pop it on the stove make sure you use oils with monosaturated fats like canola or olive oil.

Be careful with microwave popcorn. Check the labels for sodium and fat content because it varies from brand to brand.

Almonds and Other Nuts

You've heard the old phrase "An apple a day keeps the doctor away." Well now people are saying the same thing about a handful of nuts.

The biggest weapon contained in nuts is the monosaturated fat. This kind of fat is actually good for you and can even help clear your arteries.

Nuts help fill you up and are also high in Vitamin E, fiber and magnesium. Vitamin E is an antioxidant that helps fight diseases such as cancer, asthma, osteoporosis and a host of other inflammations.

Sunflower Seeds Will Also Work

Sunflower seeds are like a cousin to the nut and contain a lot of the same good characteristics. If you choose to eat these, be sure to choose the ones with low or no salt. Many people like to lick the salt from the shell and that's when a healthy snack turns into a not-so-healthy snack. The salted shells are fine in moderation but just be sure to limit your consumption.

Peanut Butter

Peanut butter is a delicious member of the legume family. It has a lot of the same good qualities as regular nuts, and is great because it will fill you up quickly. If you ever want to hold yourself over to the next meal just eat a couple of teaspoons of peanut butter. That's 190 calories right there and you get a load of protein. You can also add it to your fruit, crackers, or even a smoothie. It makes a great healthy snack.

Watch your consumption of it, however. Despite the protein, peanut butter is considered a high-calorie food. So be sure you don't overdo it.

Smoothies

Fruit smoothies can actually be used as a meal replacement if you pack them with enough ingredients. Depending upon what you put in them, they can contain anywhere between 400 and 600 calories which will keep you full for hours. The benefit to this kind of snack is you can get fruit, protein, fiber and dairy all in one delicious serving. The choice is up to you.

Note: If you're watching your sugar intake, please understand that *smoothies are very high in sugar* - even though most of it is natural.

 Sugar turns into fat when it's not burned off, so we wouldn't eat a smoothie everyday. If you really find yourself enjoying them, see if you can order a "light" or "low sugar" smoothie. Many places offer this option.

Beef Jerky

 Who knew? Beef jerky is actually a very healthy snack contrary to popular belief. On average, one ounce of jerky contains about 70-80 calories, 12 grams of protein and around 1 gram of fat. Just remember to buy your jerky at a health food store. The kind you see in regular grocery stores are generally very high in sodium.

Low Fat Yogurt

 An 8-ounce cup of yogurt generally contains 2-3 grams of fat and around 150 calories. This is a much better snack food option than something like ice cream. A recent study showed people that consumed three servings of light yogurt daily as part of a reduced-calorie diet lost about 20 percent more weight than those who only cut calories. Some recipes will even call for low fat yogurt to replace sour cream.

For Further Reading

Enjoy a healthy lifestyle and enrich your bookshelves with unbiased food and nutrition books recommended by dietitians.

Cholesterol & Heart Disease

Controlling Cholesterol the Natural Way : Eat Your Way to Better Health with New Breakthrough Food Discoveries

Dr. Kenneth H. Cooper's all-new plan to lower cholesterol without drugs! Dr. Kenneth H. Cooper, a leading authority on controlling cholesterol, shares his all-new plan for balancing your blood lipids--without drugs and without side effects. Drawing on clinical trials and the most up-to-date medical research, Dr. Cooper explains how exciting new food discoveries can give you a revolutionary new way to manage your cholesterol.

Sports Nutrition

Sports Nutrition Guidebook 3rd edition

A renowned sports nutritionist and registered dietitian shares advice she gives to athletes to enhance performance and promote good health.

This expanded edition of her best seller discusses strategies for weight control, exercise and training, avoiding eating disorders, and more. Also includes numerous recipes with nutrient analyses.

Vegetarianism

The New Becoming Vegetarian: The Essential Guide To A Healthy Vegetarian Diet

The evidence is in millions of people are moving toward a vegetarian diet because it offers a healthful and environmentally sound alternative.

Becoming Vegetarian is the ultimate source for making this valuable and beneficial life change. Packed with authoritative vegetarian nutrition information from established experts, this powerful book takes the worry out of making an important, healthy transition.

The Entrepreneur Diet

Mainstream diets, daily two-hour workouts . . . They just don't fit the lifestyles of busy entrepreneurs, or anyone who's crunched for time. If you have a daily routine that keeps you constantly on the go, you know just what we mean. That's why the publishers of Entrepreneur magazine and an advisory board of world-renowned experts in nutrition, health, exercise and goalsetting joined forces with Tom Weede to develop this groundbreaking diet and exercise plan.

Shed pounds, shape up and boost energy in just six weeks! Eat healthy without sacrificing taste or time with a six-week meal plan that offers both traditional meals and "Quick Fix" options from Starbucks, McDonald's, great restaurants and more. Start a workout plan that works with your schedule, not against it.

The Mayo Clinic Plan: 10 Steps to a Healthier Life for Everybody!

Fad diets, weight-loss gimmicks, and get fit quick exercise machines abound, but none provide lasting results. Too quickly people fall off these diets, stop using the latest machine, and lapse back into their unhealthy habits.

The clutter of diet options and conflicting advice leaves us all the more confused. Imagine if you could follow a simple, straightforward ten-step plan to a healthier life from the worlds leading medical experts? The Mayo Clinic Plan is culled from MAYO Clinic's current research and world-renowned medical experts, and includes the keys to healthy eating and a healthy lifestyle that are easy to follow. From achieving your optimal weight through eating the right foods and watching portions (and not necessarily carbs) to the incredible health benefits of incorporating exercise or any physical activity into your weekly life, the important new findings on the impact of sleep, and much more, you'll feel a difference quickly by following these steps.

The New American Heart Association Cookbook (25th Anniversary Edition)

This 25th-anniversary edition of the classic, bestselling cookbook contains 600 heart-healthy recipes, 150 of them brand-new. The book has been updated to reflect the use of nonfat and low-fat ingredients that didn't exist just a few years ago. , this book has an array of choices.

Many are healthier versions of old favorites--such as Eggplant Parmesan, Chicken ala King, Sweet and Sour Pork, Spaghetti with Meat Sauce, Devil's Food Cake, and Chocolate Chip Cookies--with some new entries that reflect modern eating trends, like Portobello Mushroom Wrap with Yogurt Curry Sauce, Pad Thai, Curried Quinoa Salad with Cranberries and Almonds, and Artichoke and Chick-Pea Pilaf. Whether you want a quick meal, a nutritious dinner the whole family will enjoy, or a festive entrée to impress guests.

Betty Crocker's Low-Fat, Low-Cholesterol Cooking Today

Not one for fads, Betty sensibly bases this 175-recipe cookbook on the Food Guide Pyramid guidelines recommended by the American Heart Association and many other medical and nutrition professional organizations. You learn tips for cutting down on fat and cholesterol, understanding the different kinds of fat, and making smart food choices for heart health.

The idea is to reduce fat by making ingredient substitutions and small alterations, but not making drastic changes. The recipes are varied and creative and don't resemble "diet food.

Low fat Cooking For Dummies

Television chef Lynn Fischer (known to many as "the Low Cholesterol Gourmet") has created a guide to low fat cooking that doubles as a crash course in home economics. In the first two parts of the book, Fischer combines basic nutrition facts with tips for establishing a "low fat" kitchen, including a guide to selecting flavorful vinegars and advice on choosing the best cuts of meat. The third (and lengthiest) part of the reference consists of more than 150 recipes that encompass every meal of the day; each recipe includes nutritional information, and many feature tips for extending or altering the meal

The American Dietetic Association's Complete Food & Nutrition Guide

Many people treat this Nutrition Guide as the "Bible", Comprehensive consumer guide includes new chapters on the use and abuse of supplements, an expanded chapter on women's health and nutrition, help for making the right food choices in restaurants, information on water and food safety, food labeling, managing body weight, and more.

In this straightforward guide to a healthy diet, Hark and Dean, nutritionists and educators both, decode the conflicting messages about nutrition that people often get from the news and from various weight-loss programs. After imparting tips on subjects like smart snacking, exercising and drinking water, they explain nutritional concepts, breaking down the food pyramid and providing a directory of vitamins and minerals.

Perhaps the most useful section describes how to "eat for the time of your life"; the authors include graphs of healthy weights, charts listing foods that are good for certain age groups and plenty of sound advice for athletes, pregnant women and people of all ages. They also demystify the main fad diets, look at how food is related to health problems and discuss buying and storing food; a handy guide to common foods' nutritional value appears at the end. Lists, questionnaires, "jargon busters" and even a few recipes are sprinkled throughout in colorful boxes, and sidebars containing case studies (i.e., a preschool child who will eat only white food) provide advice for common problems.

365 Days of Healthy Eating from the American Dietetic Association

As a health-conscious reader, you already know all about the benefits of healthy eating and active living. But some days it's harder than others to put that knowledge to good use. Smart eating and an active lifestyle should be easy and enjoyable, not a chore! Let 365 Days of Healthy Eating from the American Dietetic Association show you an easier way to start living a healthier lifestyle, one day at a time.

Bestselling author and nutrition expert Roberta Larson Duyff provides easy-to-implement hints, tips, and strategies for:
* Having a smart eating mindset.
* Making easy everyday food choices that benefit your health.
* Buying right-for-you foods and supplements.
* Preparing food for good nutrition, health, and great flavor–with easy-to-fix recipes that are as good for you as they are great-tasting.
* Getting more health and phytonutrient benefits from foods you enjoy.

The Complete Idiot's Guide to Total Nutrition (3rd Edition)

With all the constant debate over diet fads, proper nutrition is slipping through the cracks.

This revised and updated guide places the emphasis on good health by informing families of everything they need to know to get the best nutrition—from daily vitamin and mineral intake and facts about fats and cholesterol, to advice on shopping for healthy foods, and much more.

* Includes updates to the USDA's Food Guide Pyramid
* New numbers for blood pressure and sodium intake.
* A section on helping overweight children.
* New fiber recommendations for kids.
* A new section on macrobiotics and raw diets.

American Heart Association Meals in Minutes Cookbook: Over 200 All-New Quick and Easy Low-Fat Recipes

Think you don't have time to cook? WRONG! With over 200 recipes that take thirty minutes or less to prepare, you can discover the joys of cooking at home without fuss or bother.

Menu suggestions, shopping lists, and cooking tips make it a cinch to get a delicious and heart-healthy meal on the table fast.

Vegetarian Books

The New Becoming Vegetarian: The Essential Guide To A Healthy Vegetarian Diet

Comprehensive and well-researched, this new edition provides everything you need to know about making a healthy transition to a vegetarian diet or maximizing its benefits if already a vegetarian. Updated with the latest recommendations for intakes of vitamins, minerals, proteins, and fats, the authors show how to achieve optimal nutrition for all stages of life. Easy-to-read tables, figures, menus, and food guides help you determine how to meet your nutritional requirements.

You'll also learn what plant-based dietary components and factors play active roles in both the prevention and treatment of chronic illnesses.

Vegetarian Times Vegetarian Beginner's Guide

What these compilers--magazine writers--excel at is explaining, once and for all, the facts about shunning meat. Included in their discussions are different types of vegans, rebuttals of the "improper nutrition" myth, health issues from cancer to osteoporosis, alternative medicine, and environmentally friendly lifestyles.

Plain and simple language infused with appropriate humor is augmented by 14 menus with 35 recipes and shopping lists, by end-of-chapter reading lists, and by sidebars filled with information and suggestions about tofu, holiday dinners, etc.

The New Moosewood Cookbook

Since its original publication in 1977, this influential and enormously popular cookbook has been at the forefront of the revolution in American eating habits. MOOSEWOOD was listed by the New York Times as one of the top ten best-selling cookbooks of all time, and no wonder. With her sophisticated, easy-to-prepare vegetarian recipes, charming pen-and-ink drawings, hand lettering, and conversational tone, Mollie introduced millions to a more healthful, natural way of cooking. This edition preserves the major revisions and additions that Mollie made in 1992, adding 5 new recipes from Mollie's current repertoire and 16 pages of beautiful color food photography.

Simple Vegetarian

Ignoring all the simplistic stuff, however, leaves the cook with a cookbook filled with recipes pulling on the flavors of all corners of the world. Fill your pantry according to the master plan, shop wisely, plan ahead, and have at it.

This is vegetarian cooking of a sophisticated kitchen and palate (using "sophisticated" in the title would presumably scare off anyone not inclined to struggle with food). Many of the recipes

This is vegetarian cooking of a sophisticated kitchen and palate (using "sophisticated" in the title would presumably scare off anyone not inclined to struggle with food). Many of the recipes could fall out of cookbooks of various ethnic origins where a mainly vegetarian diet is the rule rather than the exception.

Other Books by Benita and Jim

Renewal

Feeling stressed? Anxious? Nervous? Learn what behaviors can feed stress and how to change these behaviors to reduce it. Learn stress management and the best ways to deal with panic attacks. Find other resources to help you cope with anxiety.
ISBN # 978-1440413347

ABC's of Goal Setting.

Ever set goals and write them down? What happened? Did you reach any of them or did you give up before you got there? Supercharge your goal setting and get ready for that satisfaction that only comes after reaching one of your goals. This book makes goal setting easy. ISBN # 978-1440419183

Life Management

Are you organized? Then you aren't the person we're looking for. If you aren't as organized as you think you should be, this is the book for you. Say goodby to clutter and let order reign. We provide clever home and family management tips.; time saving tips and more. Get help managing your life.
ISBN # 978-1440417458

You Want It When?

Are you a procrastinator? Do you put off doing things until just before they're due? Do you do your Christmas shopping on Christmas Eve? There is help for all of you right here. Learn how to break the procrastination habit.   ISBN # 978-1440417067

How Toxic Are You?

Everyone is subjected to toxins everyday. Over 80,000 at last count. Living away from the larger cities helps but not as much as you think. There are toxins in our water, our food, and in our air.   What can we do to be healthy and survive our toxic world? Does fasting or jogging help? Yes, but not enough – toxins bind to fat cells. If you are at all interesting in your and your families health, this is a must read! ISBN # 978-140425590

An Introduction To Traditional Chinese Medicine

Tired of prescriptions? of taking hundreds of pills? You've probably wondered about acupuncture and chinese medicine but were afraid to take the plunge without knowing just a little bit more about what is involved and how it could benefit you. In *An Introduction To Traditional Chinese Medicine*, Benita and Jim will explain how Acupuncture, Yoga and Qigong can help you attain and stay healthy and what system of beliefs are behind how they work.
ISBN # 978-1440424586

Coming Soon

You Were Born To Excel

This book is based on a series of classes we compiled back in June of 1998. The classes were called Human Excellence Engineering. The basic series consisted of six classes as presented in this book. Two to three weeks were spent on each class. An advanced series was planned and begun but never completed. The topics covered are: In chapter 1: New Thinking Skills; in chapter 2: Inside You; in chapter 3: Changing the Past; in chapter 4: A Brighter Today; in chapter 5: Feeling Good Again; and in chapter 6: The Future Begins Here. The classes and hence, the material in this book are a combination of NLP, Psychology and Shamanism. ISBN # (not yet assigned)

Personal Trance-formations

More than ever, researchers are concerned with the effects of mental and emotional states on an individuals health and with the possibility of treating the patient as an active and responsible participant in the healing process rather than as a passive recipient of either the disease or the cure. It is this emphasis that provides the basis for using a variety of techniques that enable non-medical persons to control pain perception and create their own response to illness. The mind plays a vital role in healing, more even than modern medicine has so far acknowledged. This guidebook to your inner world, the inner landscape of your soul, will help you connect with your most authentic feelings and thoughts. It contains a variety of techniques for dealing with this deep inner material. ISBN # (not yet assigned)

Approaching Wisdom

Storytelling is essential to the shaman's craft. There was more to the old tales than just a good yarn. Woven into the thrills and emotions were messages. The tales are the framework of the lore and the lore is a body of teachings and an essential part of the shaman's working life. Through lore we re- create the ancient strands of Otherworldly knowledge buried deep in our unconscious and bring them to the forefront of our conscious mind. We can then see them from a new perspective and apply them to life in our "everyday" world. This book recreates the shaman's storytelling as a quest for wisdom. In it we explore ways through story, myth and exercises to expand your sensory awareness, achieve internal union and contact your transpersonal self. This book provides tools, but the real exploration is up to you. ISBN # (not yet assigned)

The Castle of the Grail

The Quest for the Grail is not a fairy tale for children. It is a serious undertaking. The journey is full of trials and tribulations. The inner landscape of the Quest is full of dark forests, winding paths, narrow places, bridges, gates and castles. It is a very confusing place for us because we start foolish and ignorant. We do not recognize our guide and are frightened of what we might find. We are tested severely and ruthlessly but with mercy. The Quest is about Self Transformation and personal liberation. There is a unifying principle at the heart of all of these ways of thought, which can only be grasped by symbols, analogies and myths. Jung explained this with his archetypes of the collective unconscious. ISBN # (not yet assigned)

The Gold Mine in PLR.

What is PLR? How can it benefit you? P.L. and R. are the initial letters of Private Label Rights. PLR is merchandise or software, most of which is info or text based, customizable, and reusable as your own. The concept of PLR differs only slightly from having a ghostwriter. So if you have a website and need fresh content or are a writer and need fresh ideas - this book is a must have! ISBN # (not yet assigned)

Creativity

Would you like to be more creative? More intuitive? Would you like to learn creative problem solving? You can with the proper training. You probably already are intuitive and creative without realizing it. This book will provide the training you need to handle anything life throws at you in a more creative way.
ISBN # (not yet assigned)

Never Pay for Computer Software Again

Would you like to get a totally free operating system for your PC? How about an office suite that is rated better than Microsoft Office without Microsoft's price tag? Would you like free Image manipulation (Graphics) software? Games, Productivity software, Business applications - and all for free? How about one of the best web browsers around? Interested? It's all explained right here in Never Pay for Computer Software Again. Interested? You should be.
ISBN # (not yet assigned)

Surviving Life

How do you stay cheerful in the face of adversity, loss of job, bankruptcy, taxes and all the other things that life can throw at you?
ISBN # (not yet assigned)

Take Control (It's Your Book)

Covers everything the author needs to know about self publishing. Copyrights, ISBN numbers, writing software versus page layout software, cover design, book layout, POD versus conventional printing methods, marketing, distribution, advertising, etc. ISBN # (not yet assigned)

The Family Book of Fairy Tales

Stories of Princes and Princess's, enchanted giants and mighty ogres, lions, tailors and onions collected from around the world and assembled in this book to amuse you and your children. Includes the following stories: Cinderella's Daughter, The Giant's Hand, The Prince and the Lions, The Three Buns, The Boyer's Bride, How the Sea Became Salt, The Captive Princess, The Enchanted Oranges, The Knight of the Onion Shield, The Trade That No One Knew and The Prince and The Tailor. ISBN # (not yet assigned)

Benita's Encyclopedia of Crystals and Stones

What gems, crystals or stones have healing properties? Which do not? Which stones would you use for High Blood Pressure? Which for blood disorders? Which stones would be more effective for sores and wounds? How would you use Calcite in healing? ISBN # (not yet assigned)

Handy Order Form

Fax orders: 520-297-1293. (Send this form)

Telephone orders: 520-297-1293

(Have your credit card handy)

Email orders: Tranzform@Comcast.net <Attn. Orders>

Postal orders: Orders * 8571 N. Calle Tioga * Oro Valley, Az.

85704

Please send the following books, software or reports:
I understand that I may return any of them for a full refund for
any reason.

ISBN No. ――――――――――――――――― Quantity ☐

Title: ――――――――――――――――――

ISBN No. ――――――――――――――――― Quantity ☐

Title: ――――――――――――――――――

Name: ―――――――――――――――――

Address: ――――――――――――――――

City: ――――――――――― State :――――――― Zip: ―――――

Phone: ―――――――――――

Email: ―――――――――――――――――――――

I would like more information on other books and/ or

products ` — — — — — — — — — — — — — — — — — — ☐

  Arizona residents, please add 8.1% Sales Tax.

Handy Order Form

Fax orders: 520-297-1293. (Send this form)

Telephone orders: 520-297-1293

(Have your credit card handy)

Email orders: Tranzform@Comcast.net <Attn. Orders>

Postal orders: Orders * 8571 N. Calle Tioga * Oro Valley, Az.

85704

Please send the following books, software or reports:
I understand that I may return any of them for a full refund for
any reason.

ISBN No. _____ Quantity

Title: _____

ISBN No. _____ Quantity

Title:_____

Name: _____
Address: _____
City: _____ State :_____ Zip: _____
Phone: _____
Email: _____

I would like more information on other books and/ or

products   ------------------------------

Arizona residents, please add 8.1% Sales Tax.